The Additive Puzzle

For Andy

The Additive Puzzle

Making sense of unexplained mood/ behaviour and health problems

by Judy Bowers

Matador
9 Priory Business Park,
Wistow Road, Kibworth Beauchamp,
Leicestershire. LE8 0RX
Tel: (+44) 116 279 2299
Fax: (+44) 116 279 2277
Email: books@troubador.co.uk
Web: www.troubador.co.uk/matador

ISBN 978 1783061 365

British Library Cataloguing in Publication Data.
A catalogue record for this book is available from the British Library.

Typeset by Troubador Publishing Ltd, Leicester, UK
Printed and bound in Great Britain by
Clays Ltd, St Ives plc

Matador is an imprint of Troubador Publishing Ltd

In a Nutshell

There's a lot of information in this book, but here are the key points:

- I'm convinced that four food additives can cause mood/behavioural and health problems for some children and adults. These additives are:

E621   Monosodium glutamate (MSG)
E951   Aspartame
E950   Acesulfame K
E211   Sodium benzoate

There are six food colourings that have historically been a problem. Fortunately there has been a voluntary ban on these since 2009 in the UK, and any products that might still contain them have to print a warning on their packaging. See Chapter 4.

- At the beginning it may look daunting that you have to check labels of everything you buy, but after a couple of weeks it becomes second nature. If family life is improved it will have been well worth the effort.

- Of course there may be more additives in today's food and

drink causing behavioural and/or health problems. But by avoiding the four I list you're more likely to avoid any cocktails of questionable additives.

- You may find your child is only affected by one or two of the additives I mention. This is why doing a diary for a couple of weeks could really help.

- It really is best if the whole family can try avoiding the additives together. I have seen evidence that if a parent had behavioural problems as a child, there is a stronger chance their children will experience the same.

- 'But we don't eat junk food and have a good diet!' It may be that you just need to change your stock cubes, gravy granules and the brand of sugar-free squash you use.

- You don't need to change the type of foods you eat (unless you live off takeaways). You just need to find the makes that do not have the dubious additives in their ingredients list. These can often be cheaper, and hopefully – if life becomes easier with the behaviour of your child – you will want to introduce healthier choices.

- It's virtually impossible to avoid these additives all the time, but it's good to try and avoid the cocktail effect. For instance, if you're out for a meal and you have gravy, maybe avoid the on-tap fizzy drinks.

- To start with just try avoiding the four additives listed. You may want to explore the extended list of MSG related additives in

Chapter 4 if products with MSG in seem to have caused a problem.

- Of course not everyone is outwardly affected by the food additives I mention. But since researching for this book, and seeing some of the side effects besides behavioural problems, I personally feel these additives should be avoided by as many people as possible.

- If enough of us take action, by not buying products containing the dubious additives, my hope is that the manufacturers will have to change their ways – which will go a long way towards improving the health of our nation!

Important!

It's important to note that I don't claim that avoiding certain food additives will *automatically* help these mood/behavioural problems. If you experience any improvement where prescribed medication is involved, it's vital that you seek professional advice from your doctor/specialist before stopping any prescribed medication or treatment.

All the contributors' names have been changed.

Contents

Contents

Foreword

As a Child and Adolescent Therapist working in West Sussex for a number of years I came to know Judy and her tireless work on additives.

I worked with Sam who is mentioned in the book and noted the vast improvement, not only in his behaviour but in his self esteem and ability to apply himself at school. He was better able to work in his therapy and progressed in leaps and bounds.

In my work I came across many children who benefited from Judy's research and many family and foster placement breakdowns were avoided as a result of the adults being willing to try additive avoidance in the first instance.

In my own family a niece has been able to help her son become calmer and more sociable by rigidly keeping to an additive free diet. For my husband and I, we both react to Chinese food and much as we love it we have ceased to eat it. The after affect is just not worth the good taste.

This book is an easy to read, informative guide for parents and professionals and I am delighted that Judy has taken the brave step to have her years of work acknowledged and published.

Judy, I wish you all success with this venture and thank you on behalf of the many children that you have helped to live fuller, trouble free lives.

Elizabeth Kennedy-Finlayson BA MA CQSW
Child and Adolescent Therapist
August 2012

Introduction

The last thing I expected to be doing at this stage in my life was to be writing a book about which food additives to try and avoid. But as you read through *The Additive Puzzle* I hope you'll understand how my passion for this subject has evolved over the years, through my experience as a parent and foster carer, and how much I wish for your family's life to be improved, as mine has, through simply changing a few regular brands. A great deal of information and facts about these additives are out there, so I've packaged this information in a user-friendly way in the hope that you might try these ideas, and together we can prove conclusively that certain additives are compromising behaviour, mood and health issues in children and adults alike.

It all began with Sam.

He was a very bright, articulate, likeable 9 year old boy we knew from the special education unit that our foster son Tony also attended. We'd decided to take Sam on as a foster placement even though we knew he'd had a succession of placement breakdowns, and quickly found that while at times he'd be perfectly able to conform and behave, sometimes he'd become totally out of control, often for no particular reason.

There were times when we felt like were treading on eggshells. If we were to say the wrong thing he would go off on one and be quite abusive – at times even violent towards us. He could be very hyperactive, and got incredibly upset and disruptive if he didn't win at any games he happened to be playing, and always wanted the last 'say' in an argument. At other times he was calm and likeable, and able to do as he was asked the first time of asking.

I started to question why this behaviour seemed so erratic, and started to realise that possibly some of the things he was eating and drinking might be contributing to his mood/behaviour blips.

The turning point for us was a hot freshly-cooked barbeque-coated chicken I'd bought for lunch one sunny Sunday after church. I decided to sit outside and enjoy the sun where Sam, who had been fine in the morning, was also playing. He soon started to try and annoy me. I ignored him to start with, but by about 5pm he was really out of control – drawing on the hall walls, trying to trash his bedroom and using threatening words and actions towards us.

By 6pm he'd locked himself in the bathroom, and the duty social worker was trying to coax him out. My thoughts at the time were 'why us, why are we doing this?' Now I know why.

In sheer desperation I Googled 'behavioural problems'. I told Sam what I was looking for as I felt he also wanted to know why his behaviour could change so much, and he was really interested and looked with me. We found some research that had been done on the Isle of Wight in 2002 which showed that certain additives could have a negative effect on children's behaviour.

We started trying to buy food and drink that didn't contain the additives mentioned in the research, which wasn't quite so easy in those days as most squashes and fizzy drinks contained sodium benzoate. There were also rogue colourings in the sweets. But I discovered some things could be bought – all I had to do was switch to a different brand. Two weeks later Sam really started to be far more consistent with his behaviour. If any 'blips' occurred we could usually trace it back to something he ate or drank, and at the time I tended to buy separate squash and drinks for him, because you could only get organic without the sodium benzoate.

A few weeks later, after a couple of fairly major 'blips', we also found another additive to avoid. I was in the library and found a book that mentioned that monosodium glutamate (MSG or E621) could possibly cause headaches, depression and mood swings. It was in the mini pork pies he had every day for his lunch, in some famous brand flavoured crisps, and also in famous brand gravy granules and stock cubes. I started buying different brands for all the family for this, and it was not till some time later I realised I had done myself and my long suffering husband a favour!

We also found out, the hard way, that we had to ensure Sam ate and drank on a regular basis. A birthday meal out for me became a very traumatic experience when the meal was slow to come, and Sam hadn't eaten for hours... Need I say more?

You can imagine how thrilled Sam was to find that he had a means to control his behaviour, and over the next few months he had to unlearn some of the negative responses he had. We also needed to persuade school staff, support workers and other children to 'believe' in Sam's new-found ability to behave and conform most of the time. After nine months or so Sam was able, with some counselling and support, to go to a local mainstream primary school.

Wanting to help others, Sam designed a yellow card listing the food additives to avoid. Because it was bank card-sized it was great to take shopping, as in those days the additives were in lots of different food and drinks. I've updated the card since, to include another additive — but it's still yellow. I must have printed and laminated several hundred yellow cards over the years, and when I cut them out I always think of Sam and pray that each card will maybe help at least one child!

Sam moved on to another family after three years with us — not because of his behaviour, but because he needed to be with a younger, more active family. He continued to do well at school, joined the scouts and air cadets and did well with his GCSEs. He's now going to University, and we keep in touch by email and social network. He even popped in for tea a while ago to show us his motorbike. It's times like that that make it all worthwhile.

I look back with sadness that there were children we looked after before Sam who may have benefited from avoiding the food additives. But thanks to Sam many children, young people and families have experienced life changing results!

CHAPTER ONE

Food Additives and Me

You will have seen from Sam's story how I became interested in the affect food additives can have on children's behaviour. It was an amazing thrill to see Sam change, flourish and embrace life, but this was tinged with anger and frustration, because I could see that maybe other children and young people could be affected in the same way.

This book is designed to explain, encourage, nag and persuade people to follow my suggestions, with the hope that the result will be an improvement in their family life, relationships and/or health. I also hope that it will help provide data and evidence to make the food industry and the government sit up and take notice.

First steps in fostering

It's probably best to explain how I got involved with all these children in the first place. My husband, Paul, and I began foster caring after our own three children were 17, 14 and 12. I'd spent several years working in a special needs primary school in Worthing as a teaching assistant, before moving on to work with 16-25 year old young adults in supported housing, and then adults with mental health problems within the same organisation.

Over this time I grew to love the children and young people who somehow could not conform or behave all the time, as they were lovable rogues to me. I've also been a youth worker with different ages of children and young people at our church, and I still co-run the church parent/carer toddler group on a Wednesday.

When Paul took voluntary redundancy with the Electricity Board it seemed a natural step to combine his fantastic skills and patience as a dad with my experience with special needs and problem children. Friends in the church were foster carers with an agency, so we decided to extend the house and also become foster carers ourselves, with the same organisation.

We've had about twenty children and young people as part of our family over the years. Some stayed just for a night, some for a few weeks, several for about three years, and Tony has been with us ten years. Since he's now over 18 we've trained as adult shared lives carers for adults with special needs, so that Tony can carry on living with us until he moves on to more independent living.

Molly and George

After the amazing success with Sam, I was keen to see if other children might benefit from avoiding just a few additives, and persuading parents to simply change the brands.

I noticed George at the toddler group. He was a lovely two and a half year old boy who seemed intent on upsetting other children, and the general destruction of everything he played with. I chatted to Molly, his mum, who told me he was not like this all the time and could be very loving and kind. When I asked her what types of food and snacks he liked she was quite indignant and said 'I cook mainly from scratch'. But she used famous brand gravy and stock cubes, famous brand squash and George loved famous brand cheese and onion crisps.

And there it was. Little George was having sodium benzoate in his squash and MSG in his snacks and gravy. I gave Molly one of the yellow cards Sam had designed, and persuaded her to try avoiding these additives for a couple of weeks. Two weeks later there's one happy mum and one little boy conforming and starting to play as the other children did.

Molly was a single mum with two boys under 6, and found that avoiding the additives meant that the boys were more compliant and settling much better at bed time. But it wasn't easy for Molly to stick to avoiding the additives, as the boys would stay with their dad some weekends, and he didn't have much interest in the idea. On the following Mondays Molly's boys were having problems at school, and George would be back in destruction mode for a while.

Trust in a brand?

The initial conversation asking about which brands Molly was using became like a blueprint or script, one that I still have with parents and individuals every time there's concern over mood swings and behaviour. In virtually every conversation I have the parents say they use the famous brand gravy granules, stock cubes, certain crisps and snacks and squash, all of which still had MSG, sodium benzoate and the colourings in. At the time the voluntary ban on colours had not taken much effect, and aspartame was not in so much stuff as the 'No added sugar' campaign had only just started.

As time went on, I started to get more parents and carers interested in avoiding the dubious additives, the most interest came when the child's behaviour gave real cause for concern. As you'll see from some of the emails and stories recorded here, other parents seem quite accepting of the fact that their children's behaviour was not consistent, especially with boys.

There seems a culture of acceptance that children will misbehave and be a problem at times, and this can allow their behaviour to go unchecked for years sometimes.

Trouble in 'Middle England'

Over the past couple of years, and even more so since starting my book, I've come to realise that behaviour problems/health issues connected with food additives in children and adults alike, aren't restricted to any one 'class' or social group. In fact, it often seems to be the families that cook from scratch but use the stock cubes and gravy granules along with the famous brand squash, as they can still afford to.

An article by Laura Clark, Education Correspondent for the *Daily Mail*, in July 2012 reported a dramatic increase of violent indiscipline in primary schools. Ninety children a day are being sent home for attacking teachers and classmates. And where's this happening? Not just in deprived, backwater, underachieving schools as you might think! Apparently many of the worst cases are coming from affluent parts of the country, Teachers are reporting that spoilt middle class children are just as likely to challenge authority at school than those from less advantaged backgrounds.

Getting and giving information

Being a foster carer I've got to meet many social workers and professionals connected with children and young people. Many have taken my cards with interest, and I know certain professionals have given my cards out at a local hospital. However I rarely get feedback from this, as I now realise people need more information than what is printed on a card.

It's also true that although many people have had positive results with just avoiding these additives, there have always been some who only saw a limited amount of improvement. Since I've been writing this book I've managed to piece together more of the 'puzzle' which in some ways makes avoiding certain additives more complicated – for example MSG E621 comes in other names/forms too, which you'll see later in the book.

So I started looking at all the research that was taking place. The additives I mention have all been part of different research programmes, and I was optimistic that in as little as five years on, these additives would be removed from our foods.

Unfortunately, the different research programmes kept coming up as 'inconclusive', basically because the additives I mention have not been tested collectively and there is strong evidence that these additives are far more toxic when used together such as MSG E621 and sodium benzoate E211.

A couple of the major supermarkets seem to be taking some of the 'big four' additives and the artificial colours out of many of their products, and some have just removed a couple of the additives and colours. But you can still find them in a wide range of products.

Into the label minefield!

So where do I start to avoid these additives I hear you ask! Go through all your food cupboards, fridge and freezer and read the list of ingredients that will be somewhere on the packet or label. You'll probably be pleasantly surprised to see how much stuff is ok. When you go shopping it will take longer the first few times, but it soon becomes second nature.

Make sure you still check the products that have the reassuring ticks on the front which might say 'no artificial colours or preservatives' but may still contain artificial sweeteners aspartame, ascesuflame K or flavour enhancer MSG E621.

The famous brand flavoured crisps mostly have had the MSG removed, but not some of the snack products, so check all the crisps and snacks (especially the cheese ones that people like to give children and babies as their first grown up snack). Also beware the mini rice cake snacks, the brands specifically designed for young children are ok.

Regarding MSG E 621, initially just avoid the foods that state this on the ingredients. If you enjoy success by just doing this, it probably means you are cutting enough MSG out of your diet to make a difference. However, some people will need to use the extended list of ingredients, found in Chapter Four to identify the 'hidden' naturally occurring MSG in foods such as yeast extract.

If you see 'no added sugar' look for aspartame or acesulfame K, the famous 'blackcurrant' drinks manufacturer has a new 'No added sugar' range of different flavours with aspartame in, and very small print saying 'not recommended for children under 3'. If you're a serial 'slimmer' like myself you may well have things like sugar-free jellies etc, which usually contain aspartame. I also haven't been able to find any brand of 'no added sugar' sugar-free chewing gum without aspartame or acesulfame K. However, sucralose seems to be one of the lesser evils of the sweetener world. One of the main supermarkets uses sucralose to sweeten their drinks and does not use sodium benzoate.

As I've mentioned before, a lot of supermarket branded stuff is OK now, and you'll soon work out which supermarkets have taken these additives out of many of their products. Unfortunately, in some supermarkets you'll find it difficult to find sugar-free drinks that don't contain aspartame or acesulfame K. Basic, value and budget ranges can be fine to use too, but do check first off, and be aware some of these products may have more sugar/salt added to enhance the flavours. Maybe compare sugar and salt content with the supermarket brand versions.

The major sweet manufacturers have really cleaned up their act, as there has been a voluntary ban on adding certain colours for several years now. But do watch the cheaper brands such as candy floss and ice pops.

If you have older children and they like the 'energy' drinks, these can be a nightmare cocktail, containing the colours included in the voluntary ban. These products, by law, have to have a warning on the bottle that the product may cause hyperactivity. They can also contain high quantities of caffeine, as well as sodium benzoate to name but few.

Hopes for the future

Since gathering my material for this book I've come to realise that people do want the best for their children and themselves, and are sort of aware that additives might be a problem. But there are a couple of issues to overcome. First, we've been trained by the media and advertising industries to put our trust into certain brand names – such as famous brand gravy granules and stock cubes famous brand 'no added sugar' drinks and squashes, crisps and snacks – when in fact many of these still have the dubious additives listed in their ingredients.

Second, for the right reasons people want to do the full Jamie Oliver thing by using fresh foods and cooking everything from scratch. But some parents have experienced negative behaviour with their children when they started cooking 'from scratch' because they were using gravy granules and stock cubes which still contain the dubious additives. Initially it's probably best to keep your meals the same, just change the brands. Then, when your child is more compliant, start introducing healthier options if needed.

Something else has happened since I've been researching the affect of additives. My dear departed mother said I was a very wilful and stubborn child at times. I found it very difficult to conform and behave at school, and I tended to be the class clown, (some will say I still am). As I got older I continued to suffer from inconsistent mood swings, which I put down to having constant PMT. But about five years ago I realised that I, too, was affected by MSG E621 and aspartame – and the change in me has been immense since I have actively tried to avoid it.

CHAPTER TWO

What Are Food Additives?

The term 'food additives' applies to a range of chemicals that are added to our food, usually by the manufacturer or the producer of raw materials. The additives serve a number of purposes and fall into different categories including:

Preservatives

Improve the keeping quality and shelf-life of many products. That's why home-baked cakes don't keep as long as shop bought ones.

Colours

Colours colour things! Not all of them are bad and/or artificial – E100 comes from turmeric, which is used in some natural remedies. But many colourings have been linked with health issues in children including asthma and allergic reactions, as well as behavioural problems.

Artificial food colours such as E102 (tartrazine), E110 (sunset yellow) and ponceau red (E124) are being phased out voluntarily by the major supermarkets, sweet and food manufacturers following a report published by the UK Food Standards Agency

(FSA) in 2005. However, there are still food colourings from natural sources such as E120 (cochineal/carminic acid) which are best avoided.

Antioxidants

Another kind of preservative, antioxidants help to prevent foods with a high fat content from going rancid too quickly. You'll find antioxidants in food like sausage rolls and cooked meats.

Sweeteners

These are usually added to sweeten low-calorie products, but also in some sugar-free products for children. Artificial sweeteners are valuable to the food industry as they can be up to 200 times sweeter than sugar. Some products with sweeteners will have the letters NRC which means 'not recommended for children'

Thickeners, stabilizers, gelling agents and emulsifiers

These are added to a variety of foods for a number of reasons including ensuring ingredients don't 'split' during production. Emulsifiers help to mix water and fat, for example in mayonnaise.

Flavour enhancers

Make the taste of food stronger. The best-know flavour enhancer is monosodium glutamate, or MSG, E621 that can be found in products like crisps, Chinese food, gravy granules and stock cubes. MSG can also occur naturally in other additives which are listed in Chapter Four.

What does the E in E number mean?

An additive which has been given an E number has been approved for use within the European Union, but some are also used in the US. The problem with the E number term is that it doesn't tell us, the consumer, the shopper, which additives are natural, and which aren't.

Ethan and Dawn's story

I first met Dawn, a single mum, a year or so ago at a coffee morning. Some time later, once I'd started writing this book, we were at the same venue again. I was doing a talk about how God can come by when you least expect it, somehow (surprise, surprise) I also ended up talking about the food additives and the book.

Dawn spoke to me after and mentioned her son Ethan, aged 10. She suspected he had some sort of learning difficulty, but also had a short temper and some behavioural issues that he tended to take out on her. Sometimes he could be loving and caring, but there were tantrums and tears too. At school he seemed to be able to conform and was considered average in ability, but was very quiet, and his teachers were finally conceding that Ethan may have dyslexia or possibly dyspraxia.

Dawn felt it was as though Ethan needed to 'take it out' on her sometimes as soon as he got out of school when she picked him up. She also said he seemed to get on really well with adults, but struggled to get along with his peers sometimes.

From the start things had not been easy. Dawn suffers from Crohn's Disease and had a difficult pregnancy, partly because of all the meds she needed to treat the Crohn's. The meds affected Ethan, and from birth he had terrible colic which finally cleared up at four months. However, since then Dawn could count on one hand the times Ethan had slept through the night during his ten years.

He was also always very thirsty, and as he grew older she would give him sugar-free squash when he woke up, thinking sugar-free was better for his teeth.

I asked Dawn all the usual questions: which brand of squash, crisps, gravy granules etc they had? Apparently Ethan is a very fussy eater and would only eat dry food, so the gravy's not to blame. But he only liked the famous brand peach 'no added sugar squash' and often had crisps and snacks that had MSG in. I gave Dawn a yellow card and a leaflet, advised her to only offer water in the night, and that there was no need to tell Ethan just yet what she was doing. I also mentioned omega 3 fish oils may help too.

I caught up with Dawn about a month later, and she told me there'd been a marked change in Ethan's behaviour – he seemed a lot more confident and less tearful. She had changed the squash he drinks to a peach supermarket own brand without aspartame or sodium benzoate, and only bought him crisps and snacks without MSG. She told Ethan that she was trying to be healthier for her crones. She also started Ethan on omega 3 fish oils, and is thrilled she can now give him medicine without him having a tantrum.

Now, if Ethan gets frustrated or upset she can calm him down easily by putting strategies in place – something she couldn't do before. Also, Dawn has started to feel the benefit from avoiding the dubious additives. She's calmer too, and feels 'in control'.

Probably the most exciting thing is that Ethan is sleeping much better.

Ethan had experienced stomach ache on and off over the years. This greatly concerned Dawn as she didn't want Ethan to develop Crohn's as she had had. But since starting the new way of eating to date Ethan has had virtually no stomach problems.

CHAPTER THREE

What Is Bad/Negative Behaviour?

Of course not all negative behaviour can be blamed on various food additives. Some children may have an attachment disorder (through lack of appropriate bonding in the first few weeks of their lives), or suffered childhood trauma such as going into care or bereavement. Some may have a specific learning difficulty such as autism or dyspraxia, or possibly received diagnoses of ADHD (Attention Deficit Hyperactive Disorder), to name but few!

What I've found with these behaviours, especially ADHD, is that the behaviour is often consistent regardless of circumstance and time of day. However, the outcomes of even these behavioural problems may well be helped (or maybe I should say made more manageable) by avoiding the additives mentioned in Chapter Three of this book.

This 'list' has evolved over the last nine years, and is gleaned from personal experience of children we have fostered, plus information and feedback from the parents/carers of children, and in some cases adults, who have tried avoiding the additives. I'd say that probably the main indicator that a child can be helped by the method I suggest is that they may well be able to conform perfectly well at times, and others are unable to.

Specifically these are some of the behaviours and actions

of a child/young person that indicates that they may benefit from avoiding the dubious food additives:

- As a parent/carer, at times you'll have the general feeling that you are treading on 'eggshells': that if you were to say the wrong thing s/he will go off on one.

- The child doesn't understand why they behave like they do at times, and probably don't like it, but are unable to control it.

- Addiction to certain foods/flavours/brands can reveal a reaction to a particular additive.

- The child may be a fussy eater and/or be poor at drinking enough fluids. Or they can be an excessive eater, craving food and drink that have the dubious additives in.

- Moody, aggressive, stroppy, depressed, argumentative – outside the normal hormonal mood swings you'd expect from a teenager or adolescent.

- At times not willing to conform to simple everyday requests such as hand washing /brushing teeth.

- Dominating other children in play, unwilling to play games for fear of not winning.

- Sometimes you dislike your child's behaviour because of the way s/he behaves towards you, and then other times s/he would be absolutely fine.

- Difficulty in concentrating.

- Your child might be extremely likeable, lovable and caring at times, and quite able to conform, and at others seemingly not bothered or even able to try sanctions or strategies to help their behaviour. Boys especially get the nickname from teachers etc as the 'lovable rogue'.

- When starting to mix with other toddlers and children, your child might be the one that other parents don't want their children to play with.

- The home school book may say 'managed to stay in class and work this morning, but was unable to behave and played up this afternoon'.

- The problems seem to start when a child starts having the same food/snacks/drinks as the rest of the family (as foods specifically formulated for babies and toddlers do not have the rogue additives in).

- Your child may have unexplained health issues like stomach ache after drinking sugar-free drinks with added sweeteners.

- Your baby/child may become hyperactive after bath time and find it difficult to settle at night.

- In extreme cases you may experience violent aggressive behaviour towards yourselves and others which can be very difficult to deal with.

- Teachers or professionals may suggest having your child assessed for ADHD, however your child does not 'fit' the diagnosis as they do not have consistent behaviour problems.

- Children that are diagnosed with Asperger's Syndrome or autism seem more likely to be intolerant to certain food additives.

- A child may have low self esteem/and be desperate for praise from the important adults in his/her life. *(See section on 'unlearning' behaviours)*

- Your child does not seem to cope with 'life changes' as well as other children do, for instance why are some children absolutely fine when a younger sibling comes along, and some are not?

Jane's email

I met Jane at the toddler group. She also came along to other meetings we had at the church, and over time we became friends, she has three lovely children, but I noticed she and her husband seemed to have very short fuses sometimes, and her eldest daughter, who started having her periods at a very early age, seemed to have excessive mood swings and unnatural behaviours around the time before her periods. I suggested to Jane that she try avoiding the additives with all the family. This is what she had to say:

I would like to personally thank you for handing me one of your additives information card last year.

I have three children, all of whom seemed to behave relatively well most of the time. I was concerned about my husband's moods and, to be quite honest, my own too. So I decided to give the information the benefit of the doubt. I changed the supermarket I shop in, it was surprisingly cheaper than I thought! We tried to stick to non-branded food for cost effectiveness, and knowing they have removed most of these additives from their goods, I found mainly the gravy granules, crisps, snacks and squash were things I needed to change.

It has made a remarkable difference to our moods, outlook and calmness within our household. I have also noticed a positive difference in my hormonal young daughter. I would strongly recommend anyone to have a go for a few weeks. There is nothing to lose and everything to gain.

Jane

CHAPTER FOUR

The Big Four and How to Avoid them

When I started looking in to the effects of food additives on behaviour, it was obvious fairly quickly which were the main culprits. The first two I discovered were:

E621 Monosodium glutamate (MSG) – flavour enhancer
E211 Sodium benzoate – Preservative

And then about four years ago I identified:

E951 Aspartame – sweetener

And even more recently:

E950 Acesulfame K – sweetener

Which often seems to replace aspartame because of all the bad press it has received.

When we first started nine years ago there were four artificial colours as well

E102 Tartrazine
E110 Sunset yellow

E122 Carmiosine

E124 Ponceau 4R

Thankfully there is a voluntary ban on these four colourings, upheld by most of the major manufacturers. But remember they can crop up in energy drinks and very cheap sweets, drinks and ice pops.

It is important to note that you may only find one or two additives that actually seem to affect your child's behaviour – it is often about avoiding the cocktail effect!

It can be quite useful to write a food diary for the first couple of weeks which may help you identify any additives you need to leave out of your diet.

E621 Monosodium Glutamate (MSG)

What is it?

MSG is a flavour enhance that was originally discovered by the Japanese in the early 1900's, when it was formulated from seaweed. In the second world war it was used to flavour the Japanese troops' food, and its taste was known as 'umami' which roughly translates as 'savoury'. It is now formulated from monosodium salt of glutamic acid, and may be GM (genetically modified).

Where is it used?

MSG is in some fast foods, snacks/crisps, processed meat products (salami sticks) gravy granules, stock cubes, savoury rice cakes and Chinese/Japanese food, some instant flavoured noodle snacks, soy sauce, some quick soups etc.

In 1970 MSG was banned from use in baby food and is now

banned in children's food for under 3 year olds. But this doesn't apply to 'adult' food that are often eaten by children from as young as 12 to 18 months.

When starting this book my hope was to keep my ideas simple and achievable for parents and carers. Many have found that just avoiding foods that state MSG E621 on the label has worked well, so historically I have just mentioned this. The outcome of positive results seems to coincide with avoiding the 'cocktail' element with other additives that often seems the key issue.

I do feel it's important that at the start you just try avoiding foods that have MSG as a listed ingredient, not this extended list. Many find just reducing the amount of MSG in the diet can make all the difference. However, MSG can come in the guise of other names and can be 'naturally occurring' in many processed foods, for example:

- Hydrolyzed vegetable protein

- Monopotassium glutamate (any protein that is hydrolyzed)

- Glutamic acid

- Yeast extract

- Sodium caseinate

- Autolyzed yeast extract

The following very OFTEN contain MSG:

- Malt extract flavours(s) and flavouring(s)

- Bouillon – natural beef flavouring

- Stock – natural chicken flavouring

- Soy sauce/soy sauce extract

- Maltodextrin

- Whey protein/whey protein isolate/whey protein concentrate

- Soy protein/soy protein isolate/soy protein concentrate

Brands with 'No MSG' are OK to use, but beware of products that claim 'no added MSG' as they may well have dubious flavour enhancers under different names included. If you feel the need to research this further there is plenty of information on sites such as MSGTruth.org

Why/how does MSG cause a problem?
MSG has actually been used in our food for years, but it's only recently that its reported negative effects have become apparent. This is interesting if you compare its effects in Japan and China, where MSG is used in large quantities. In these countries people still seem to cope without ill effect, and it seems to be down to the fact that they eat far more fresh food

than we do and eat smaller portions. They also probably have less of the other dubious additives so they are not subjecting themselves to a questionable cocktail.

This also goes some way to explain why we seem to be more affected by MSG these days. Historically, our diet was three meals a day with virtually no snacks or fast food – and again people weren't subjected to today's 'cocktail' of additives.

There are also cultural issues. It used to be that even if a child/young person was affected by MSG there was a culture of 'expectation' regarding behaviour in school and the home. And in Japan and China children are still expected to behave and conform in a certain way.

How can behaviour be improved through avoiding MSG?

Donna's story – written with Donna

I met Donna at our toddler group in 2005. She started coming with her middle child and her new baby. Her oldest child, Katy, was already at school. The time came for Donna's youngest child to go to preschool, and as Donna needed to get some work experience, she stayed on as a volunteer to do craft activities with the children.

As we got to know Donna it became obvious that things were not entirely 'happy' at home with her family life, and as the children got older things became worse, which caused problems in her marriage. The main problem seemed to be Katy and her attitude towards Donna at home, which resulted in Katy being shipped off to her grandparents for several weeks as they couldn't get on. It was on the cards that Donna and her husband would split up and Donna wanted Katy to go and live with her dad.

In many ways I could see aspects of myself in Katy's behaviour. In particular how I'd been with my attitude and mood swings, before I discovered that I needed to avoid MSG, so I mentioned the food additive idea several times to Donna. She wasn't really interested, and so this went on for a couple of years.

Then one Monday I read on Donna's social network page CAN MY LIFE GET ANY WORSE! I was determined that this time she'd listen to me. I tackled her at the next toddler group, and she finally agreed to look at what Katy was eating and drinking for a couple of weeks. She told me she daren't tell Katy what she was doing and she didn't. Katy complained bitterly and very verbally about the change to supermarket own brand crisps, no salami sticks and cheaper non-brand sugar-free squash, but Donna just said she was trying to cut the housekeeping budget a bit.

After a week or so Donna conceded that things did seem to be getting better, although their relationship was still quite strained. I started to talk through with Donna how she needed to start believing in Katy and 'allow' and 'give permission' for Katy to behave.

I took Katy out for breakfast one day and explained to her about the additive situation, and how her Mum was trying to avoid the additives in her diet. Katy was really pleased and could see that she was in fact coping better with life. She was also keen to learn how to 'unlearn' some of her behaviours, so over the next few weeks I acted as a bit of a mediator between Donna and Katy, which helped them start to appreciate and understand each other and the rest of the family.

Katy had not really been a problem at school and was doing quite well, although she did struggle with maintaining friendships. She got praise from school when she did well, and was craving praise from Donna who felt she could rarely give it as it was not deserved.

Things started to look up for the family, but as far as Donna was concerned the main problem had been Katy and the additives. One Monday Donna's social network page read I HATE MONDAYS LIFE IS ****. I posted the comment 'so what did you have to eat over the weekend? Was it Chinese or good old famous brand gravy granules?' It had been Chinese on the Saturday, and gravy at her mum's on the Sunday. By the Wednesday Donna had finally conceded that the whole family needed to avoid the additives where possible, including her husband who was still having famous brand vegetarian gravy, and stock cubes.

These days things have gone from strength to strength for Donna and her family. They have even had a couple of holidays together, which would not have happened before. Donna and Katy are good friends now and enjoy spending 'special' time together.

How can I avoid MSG?

- Check the label! Avoid any food which contains monosodium glutamate or MSG E621. It's also an option to avoid anything the extended list as mentioned before.

- Supermarket own-brands are more likely to be MSG-free than branded foods, but don't forget to check.

- If the label just says the food contains 'flavouring' or 'flavour enhancer' it could well be MSG.

E951 Aspartame

Aspartame didn't really come under my radar until four or five year ago.

Although MSG, sodium benzoate and the four food colours seem to be slowly being taken out of our food and drink, aspartame is going from strength to strength due to the incredible increase of diet-related food and drink. There are two reasons for this. First, since 2002 the World Health Organisation (WHO) has been putting pressure on the food industry to reduce the sugar and fat content in our foods in an effort to combat the obesity epidemic. Second, the food industry has been trying to meet consumers' growing desire for 'no added sugar' products.

Think about the 'tooth friendly' squashes, many of which are now 'double-concentrate' (hands up those who do not halve the amount they use), the ever-increasing range of 'sugar-free' chewing gum and sweets, and top it off with those who are 'addicted' to famous brand diet cola drinks. Houston we have a problem!

Since people I've talked to have been avoiding this with their children and for themselves there have been many pleasing results reported – not only regarding behaviour, but also health issues like acid reflux, migraine, stomach aches and other problems to name but few. Although late to join the Judy B quest to identify an easy way to avoid dodgy additives – and after looking at the research available – this is now one of the main contenders for avoidance.

Elena's email

I met Elena, a lovely young Spanish mum, at the toddler group. I had been handing out my leaflets, and got chatting about the additives as I do.

Hi Judy

It was good to see you yesterday and talk about what happened to me about a year and a half ago.

It all started when I was about seven months pregnant with my child. I suddenly had a craving for chewing gum and obviously my first choice was to buy a 'sugar-free' well known brand. I never did pay any attention to the ingredients, I just noticed a warning on the package saying that too many chewing gums can have a laxative effect.

However, as the months passed by, I got addicted to them and every time the flavour disappeared I had an urgent need to take another one. It got to a point that I consumed about two packets per day, an equivalent to 20 more or less.

I remember starting in the morning just after having breakfast and I would carry on until bed time. I never thought there was something wrong with it, but everyone around me told me that I had become addicted to them.

When my son was about four months old I had to go to Spain, and spent about seven months on my own due to the building work being carried out in our house in Lancing.

I remember vividly how I was chewing all the time and sometimes I could feel my heart beating faster than usual. I had terrible swing moods, which I never had had before. I got really agitated for anything and did not have any patience at all. At the time I did assume that I was really stressed and never in a million years linked that change in my character with the consumption of chewing gum which contains aspartame amongst other additives.

I have always being aware of additives in food and always do check the labels. I cook mostly everyday from scratch and try to provide well balance and healthy meals for my family. For instance, I never buy fruit juices with aspartame for my children. I'd rather give them juice with added sugar.

Ironically, my daily intake of aspartame through the consumption of chewing gum was immense and even today I think back of that period of my life with great sadness and regret. That person wasn't me and my children had to suffer my swing moods for all that time.

When I met you at the playgroup you run at the Tabernacle and gave me that list with the additives and information, 'something clicked in my head'. I decided to stop eating chewing gum for good and I can proudly say that I have come back to my old self and have not tried them for months.

I realise there is nothing I can do about that past period in my life now. However if this story could help to give awareness of the dangers of additives, in my case aspartame, something positive would come out from it.

Amazingly, even today when I go to the supermarket and stand next to the till I still feel tempted to buy chewing gum. Also, when I brush my teeth, I instantly think of chewing gum as the toothpaste has also got aspartame in its composition!

Judy, I think you are doing an amazing job making people aware of the dangers of additives. Keep going and thank you very much!

See you soon.

Best Wishes, Elena

What is it?

Aspartame is an artificial sweetener. It was discovered by accident in 1965 by a chemist who worked at GD Searle & Co. He was testing an anti-ulcer drug and found it had a sweet taste that was 200 times sweeter than refined sugar.

If you were to look at a website, such as www.healthychoices.co.uk/aspartame, you'll see the history of controversy that has taken place about this additive, and the effect it can have on children and adults alike. America is shouting louder than us because there seems more evidence about the adverse effects – mainly due to the fact that they have had aspartame in their diets for much longer than us. Over 75% of adverse reactions to food additives reported to the US Food and Drug Administration (FDA) were due to aspartame.

In the UK, aspartame was first approved for general consumption in 1982. Despite many case studies and anecdotal reports, research into aspartame is often deemed 'inconclusive'. I believe this is because it isn't tested alongside sodium benzoate or MSG.

Since I first started 'doing my thing' and discovering certain additives did cause behavioural/health problems, I was reassured in some ways to see that many brands had started to exclude the MSG and sodium benzoate. So whilst we have seen some very positive results in that time, since I've started to mention excluding aspartame as well results have been even better and more consistent. But it wasn't until I started gathering my evidence for the book that I realised the huge scale of the aspartame empire.

Where is it used?

In all kinds of food and drinks which need sweetening,

particularly products labelled 'sugar-free'. Often mixed with acesulfame K (see below).

Is it known by any other name?
Not that I'm aware of at the moment, but be aware that some major brands of artificial sweeteners are made of aspartame.

Why/how does aspartame cause a problem?
Some of the bad reactions reported to the US Food and Drug Administration (FDA) include:

- Headaches/migraines
- Muscle spasms
- Weight gain
- Acid reflux
- Depression
- Insomnia
- Vision problems
- Hearing loss
- Tinnitus
- Memory loss
- Heart palpitations
- Loss of appetite
- Joint pain
- Asthma

Studies have also indicated that aspartame can trigger or worsen:

- Brain tumours
- Multiple sclerosis

- Epilepsy
- Chronic fatigue syndrome
- Parkinson's disease
- Alzheimers
- Birth defects
- Fibromyalgia
- Diabetes
- Certain types of cancer

In July 2010 EU funded research by Danish scientists looked at nearly 60,000 mothers to be, and found there was a link between the amount of diet drinks consumed and early birth. Prior to that the independent Ramazzini Foundation in Italy published research suggesting aspartame caused several types of cancer in rats at doses very close to the acceptable daily intake for humans.

This concerns me greatly with the advent of double-concentrate squash, many individuals being 'addicted' to diet coke, and the ever increasing list of food and drink that is containing aspartame. Both of these research cases were evaluated by European Food Standards Agency (EFSA) experts who rejected any risk to human health.

How can behaviour be improved through avoiding aspartame?

Liam's story

I was at a slimming club (my second home) 3 years ago when I overheard a mum talking about her then six year old child. She was saying she couldn't leave him alone with her new baby as she couldn't trust his behaviour, and that his behaviour also meant he was struggling at school. I went into interfering mode and spoke to Linda asking her my stock questions such as *does he act like this all the time?* she said that no, sometimes he was fine and very loving. I mentioned the food additives and gave her a yellow card. I also told her I was starting to realise aspartame was starting to be an issue, so she took that one on board too.

A few weeks after she started doing it I emailed Linda to see how she was getting on, and this is the response I got in September 2009:

Hi Judy,

Thanks for sending all the information through – I found it all very useful, and the first thing I did was to check everything that he eats already for the additives.

Although I didn't find a huge amount containing the named additives, I was able to identify a few which he would take to school in his lunch box – that might explain why the school was reporting behaviour being considerably worse in the afternoons than the mornings! The two items I've stopped are some famous brand scary snacks (contained MSG) and famous make lunch box drink – contained aspartame – (this brand has now changed the sweetener in this product to ascesuflame K) although this wasn't on your list, we just talked about it.

I have also upped his omega 3 intake so he has 2 of the ******* omega 3 gums. Liam did start back at school a lot more settled, but the last week or so he is even more noticeably different. He previously hated PE and sports and has now joined the tennis club at school and loves it – I was a bit worried as at the end of last term he was throwing tennis rackets at children, but the Coach said he was absolutely fine! I popped in to watch the last few minutes and it was wonderful to see him running around, laughing and really enjoying himself!

Liam also would resist doing his homework and it was a real battle which often ended in tantrums and crying and the work not being done. This week, however, Liam was keener to try it and even said 'It's easy peasey'. He completed the work easily and felt very proud of himself afterwards. Liam has also gone up a reading book and is now one away from going onto bigger chapter books which he is really pushing for.

The school have only got positive things to say about him at the moment and he is doing really well. I have noticed as well that the other children who previously didn't really get involved with him are now talking to him and he is being involved in discussions about the latest craze, swapping cards with them etc.

I'm not sure whether the withdrawal of just a couple of items of food or the larger intake of omega 3 is having this effect in this short period of time but we are certainly enjoying the results!

Linda

When starting to write this book I emailed Linda again to see how they were getting on. This was her update in March 2012:

Liam is getting on really well BUT I do stick to the ideas you advised me on!

We have cut out aspartame completely as if we don't he

is violently sick, so therefore he's also very good at not having things he doesn't know are clear of it, as he obviously doesn't want to get ill!

On the odd occasions when it has slipped through we have an 'unexplained' bout of sudden vomiting which is usually only the one occasion, but literally a complete clear out – excuse the gross detail! We have also found MSG can cause this as well especially if it's in conjunction with aspartame – Liam had Chinese Chicken Balls once and a diet cola drink, and then within two hours had horrendous stomach pains and dizziness which ended in him throwing up the once and then he was fine so I know it wasn't a bug.

If he eats anything with MSG in it we tend to get a dip in behaviour – usually hyperactive and disobedience, hence we have also cut this from his diet. If his behaviour suddenly goes AWOL we review what he has been eating and it will usually be something with MSG in it – like I mentioned above this can also cause stomach problems but not as severe as aspartame.

We still give him double dose of omega 3 vitamins and again if we run out and he doesn't have them there is a noticeable change in behaviour – a dip in motivation and overall 'happiness'.

Liam moved a new school in September 2010 and struggled initially, but now is average in his school work – he still finds literacy challenging but that goes hand in hand with a speech delay and his difficulties – he is coping wonderfully and making good progress in Maths and has recently joined the library and loves reading!! He can read 4 books in a week and he tells us what they are about so we know he is understanding them too. Liam attends an after school club where he fits in beautifully, *goes to after school football club and has many friends so his social skills are really improving. He also went away with the school on an Adventure 3 days last year and found it no problem which I never thought he could do.*

I would be really happy for you to use Liam as an example in your book – you have helped us immensely!! I get so cross when I can't buy squash in my local supermarket that doesn't contain aspartame, and I think it's criminal they can sell something that's so dangerous!

The pointers you gave us coincided with Liam's change in behaviour, so I firmly believe in what you do and I know what to look for if there is any change in Liam's behaviour – I would never have connected the aspartame issue if it wasn't for your advice, and you have saved us unexplained bouts of sickness which rarely occur now and if it does it's a bug that has been contracted normally. The omega 3 also has an impact as we recognise now when he isn't taking them and his thirst for learning and applying himself greatly improves when he is regularly taking the vitamins.

Thank you again for your advice and good luck with your book – so many people need to know these things!

Linda

But it's important to know that aspartame isn't just having a bad effect on some children. It can cause all kinds of problems for adults too.

How can I avoid aspartame?
This does seem to be the worst additive to avoid now, but after a couple of weeks shopping you will know by second nature what you can and can't buy.

- Aspartame is now the main sweetener for 'no added sugar' drinks even some flavoured waters. Also look out for this in sugar-free jellies, desserts, yoghurts, sweets, squashes, fizzy drinks, table top sweeteners and tablets, sauces, sugar-free chewing gum.

- As I have mentioned before, two supermarkets have taken this sweetener out most of their products, however beware of acesulfame K that can sometimes be used as a replacement. You will also need to avoid famous brand and other brands of 'no added sugar' squash. The famous blackcurrant cordial company has recently bought out a range of 'no added sugar' fruit drinks with aspartame in, but the small print says not recommended for children under three. Often the best option in your supermarket may be the high juice (but not the 'no added sugar' one).

- When you go through your cupboards/fridge/freezer initially you may be able to work out if the supermarket you shop in still has aspartame in their products.

- Be very aware of the 'this is safe to buy' tick list.

- Famous brand 'lunch box' bottles of 'no added sugar' squash has had the aspartame taken out and replaced with acesulfame K.

- Look out for aspartame in oral care products and sugar-free chewing gum.

Shirley's email

I met Shirley at a Parent Factor group meeting recently where I talked about guess what!

Hi Judy,

As promised here goes!!

A brief introduction: we are a 'normal' family of five, my husband, myself, Tim (13), Ann (8) and Elsie (6).

I have always been stroppy/tearful around about the week before my periods, often had headaches and had very sore knees (doc says wear and tear!). And like lots of people I also wanted to lose some weight, so was living on diet drinks, sugar-free yoghurts, sweeteners in my coffee etc.

Tim – has suffered from bedwetting since he was 6 years old (on medication for this) has specific literacy and numeracy difficulties, poor organisational skills, finds it hard to set to task and harder still to stay on task! He also has headaches.

Ann – quiet, loves school, only problem is headaches. Had her eyes tested, but they're fine.

Elsie – well, she is 'lively' – loves to be the clown and make people laugh, is bright but as teachers in the past have said 'am sure she has more to give'. Does what is asked then off to play, doesn't like to sit still for too long.

This was our family life till I went to Parent Factor at our school. Yes, we had boundaries – good. Yes, I shouted – not so good!

Diet? Great, so I thought – lots of healthy home made dinners, roasts, sugar-free drinks, sugar-free yoghurts etc –

not so good, I find out. Try cutting out aspartame, sodium benzoate and MSG.

Well, what can I say? The longer we've done this, the better we all are:

Me – I eat and drink full fat foods, forgot about the diet and resigned myself to the fact I need to exercise (I still haven't started). My knees no longer hurt, (they occasionally ache) I no longer have regular headaches, I don't have mood swings before my periods and I'm slowly losing weight?!!

Tim – he now gets up and dressed in the morning without me having to tell him step by step, his teachers at our recent review said that everyone has noticed how he has improved, become more independent and will now start a task rather than wait to be told to.

An even bigger thing is he has stopped bed wetting, which coincided with the time I eliminated the nasty additives, and is now only taking 1 tablet at night (he used to be on 2 different types). I don't know if bed wetting is linked to these additives, maybe something to look into – please let me know if you find a link. He also no longer gets regular headaches.

Ann – still great! She no longer complains of headaches at home.

Elsie – Her teacher told me the other week how Elsie has suddenly got an appetite to learn, she has turned into a sponge and even wanted to sit and carry on with her maths instead of going out to play?!!

All the above from changing just a few things. The crisps we buy are now cheaper lol, the drinks don't have sweeteners in and they can still have fizzy for a treat as there are some

*that don't have the nasties in. I have learnt to stay away from
'sugar-free' items.*

*If you have any other questions or find a link to the bed
wetting please let me know,*
cheers,

Shirley

What sweeteners are best to go for?

From feedback I've received, and evidence from research,
sucralose seems one of the lesser evils, and at least one
supermarket uses this as their sweetener in 'no added sugar
products'. You can also buy sucralose in powder form and tablets,
although I do feel sweeteners should be used with a great deal
of moderation in a child's diet. A table-top/baking sweetener
made from Stevia leaves is also available, but only as a
sweetener, as to date it hasn't been passed to be used in food
and drink products as manufacturers are having to test them. In
addition there's Xylitol, which also comes from a plant source.

Josh's story

Written with Abigail – his Mum:

*Abigail came as a volunteer to our toddler group. She was a
single mother, with an 8 year old son, Josh.*

*At the age of four Josh started to become unwell, with a
seemingly difficult to diagnose condition. He was having
great difficulty in walking, and his joints would become
inflamed and sore. After many trips to and fro to the doctors,
and after various blood tests, there was still no diagnosis. On*

a particularly bad day for Josh – when he couldn't move and was in so much pain he ended up in the A & E department at our local hospital – Abigail declared she wouldn't leave until they could identify what was making Josh so ill. Ten days later they left the hospital with anti-inflammatory medication, and a diagnosis of Juvenile Arthritis.

Abigail was also given a list of foods to avoid such as tomatoes, citrus fruits, red meat, and any acid fruits such as grapes and plums. The list also mentioned avoid aspartame.

This didn't mean a lot to Abigail, as she didn't really know what it was in and used for (these days it has a lot higher profile). And although she avoided the foods suggested, and aspartame in some of the foods she found it in, she didn't really see a great deal of improvement from this.

The next four years proved a testing time for Abigail and Josh. Often Josh would need to use a wheel chair to get around for a day or two, sometimes for weeks.

When Abigail started helping at Toddler group she mentioned Josh and his arthritis. I asked if she was aware certain food and fruits can aggravate the condition, she replied she was aware, and had been told to avoid aspartame too, I mentioned my work with avoiding additives. I suggested it might be good to also avoid monosodium glutamate and sodium benzoate for a couple of weeks, which she did.

In just a couple of days Abigail saw a great deal of improvement in Josh's condition, and after a week he was virtually clear of all symptoms. The only times he got any symptoms back was when he might have had one or two of the dubious additives, mainly when the special offers were

40

irresistible. She found that maybe a few bags of crisps with MSG in over a few days might be ok, but it built up, so if he had something with them that had aspartame or sodium benzoate in too (often in the lunchbox), his joints would quickly become very inflamed and stiff. They also soon learnt that when Josh's 'flare ups' occurred they could usually look back and identify one or two dubious additives that had crept in, or they had been out somewhere to eat.

When discussing the additive issue with Abigail she admitted 'aspartame' had been just a word and didn't mean much, and felt if it was allowed in foods it must be ok. She'd always tried to buy the best brands of foods such as famous brand gravy granules and famous brand squash (which in fact contained the dubious additives) for Josh, as she felt they would be better for him. Josh has never really had behavioural problems, so they found it easy to 'forget' to check everything all the time, and they found it quite difficult avoiding aspartame especially as it is in so much these days. Abigail felt lunch boxes were the most difficult to cater for.

But at the age of about eight and a half Josh was discharged from the hospital clinic, but could go back if needed. So far there's been no need to return, as Josh continues to do well and the doctors were extremely pleased and impressed with his progress. They'd previously stated that at the age of ten Josh might 'grow out of' arthritis, or it might carry on into adulthood. Josh has just had his tenth birthday, but has been virtually clear of his arthritis for a year and a half.

Abigail also mentioned she does sometimes tell other parents about the additives, but found that unless a child was

41

really causing big problems, they were not really interested.
She feels there is a culture of parents accepting their child
has behaviour issues sometime, and you just learn to live
with it.

E950 Acesulfame K

What is it?
Acesulfame K is an artificial sweetener made from synthetic chemicals similar to aspartame and is sometimes blended with aspartame.

Where is it used?
In much the same products as aspartame, and is being used to replace aspartame in some drinks etc (for instance in the famous brand lunchbox bottles of 'no added sugar' squash), probably because of the bad press aspartame is getting.

Why/how does acesulfame K cause a problem?
When tested on animals it caused lung tumours, breast tumours, leukaemia, respiratory disease and cancer. I have less evidence that acesulfame has the same effect on children's' behaviour as aspartame does, but the possible health risks alone give a good reason to avoid it. Also, it's sometimes blended with aspartame.

How can health/ behaviour be improved through avoiding acesulfame K?
Georgina is a volunteer at the toddler group, and guess what we got talking about ?

Georgina's story

Hi, my name is Georgina and I am 20. For the last ten months or so and I have had trouble with really bad acid reflux. My doctor could not find anything wrong and gave me antacids to treat the symptoms.

I did not know anything about additives but I was drinking from one to two litres of a famous brand diet cola every day. I did not connect my acid reflux to the diet cola until I started volunteering at a local mums and toddlers group.

Judy, one of the leaders, was talking about food additives and how they could affect people. I asked about aspartame because my dad had mentioned that it can cause health problems, and I wondered if it could help acid reflux. Judy said she was not sure if avoiding certain additives would help but suggested I try giving up the diet Cola for a couple of weeks to see if that made any difference.

I decided to switch to the full sugar version of the diet cola I had been drinking; within three weeks of doing that my acid reflux was completely gone. It was not easy to keep from drinking the cola I had been drinking before; I still wanted it because nothing else tasted as good to me.

I discovered that acesulfame K also gave me acid reflux when I bought a sports drink after going to the gym. I was too thirsty to check the label for additives. Two hours later I had really bad acid reflux. I looked at the ingredients on the label and found the sweetener acesulfame K listed there.

I have since been very careful to avoid both aspartame and acesulfame K and my acid reflux has not come back. While not drinking those diet drinks is difficult because I love the taste of them, avoiding the additives is as simple as switching to the full sugar versions and reminding myself that I do not want acid reflux later.

How can I avoid acesulfame K?
The same way as avoiding aspartame.

Sugar
When talking to parents and carers I'm often asked if drinks containing sugar are better for children than those containing sweeteners. Sugar has had some pretty bad press recently – I've been looking at various media and research that has taken place over the last few years, and here's my interpretation:

The early 1970s saw the advent of the diet industry with the start of the 'low-fat foods' craze. Unfortunately, unbeknown to consumers, lots of sugar was added to many of these products to keep the flavour palatable. The 70s was also the beginning of the snack era, where snacking on things like chocolate and crisps started to become the norm – as in the old 'a finger of fudge is just enough to give your kids a treat', and the one that would not spoil your appetite!

Artificial sweeteners such as saccharin started to be standard use for anyone trying to lose weight and 'diet'.

Over the decades the food industry has played with our taste buds/receptors, and our bodies are now in crisis saying to us 'make your mind up – are you giving me sugar or sweetener? And if you plan on sweetener, I'll then crave sugar as you're giving my brain the wrong information'. This, I believe, may lead to people having unnatural 'sugar cravings'.

Professor of Marketing from Harvard University Pierre Chandon talks about 'low-fat food, high fat people.' He calls it the 'halo effect' or the 'health halo.' When we have something low sugar or low calorie we then feel we can eat more of it, and maybe have something as a treat to reward ourselves for being 'good' – thus eating more than we normally would have.

He did a trial with M&M sweets. Some were labelled low-fat, and others were the original product, which people were allowed to eat freely over the course of the trial. The results showed people were eating at least 50% more of the low-fat version than the original product, so probably ending up eating the same amount of calories than a 'normal' amount of the original product. (Hands up if you have done this, I have been perfecting the art for some years now!)

If you look at many other countries that don't seem to have the obesity problems that we see in the UK and USA, sugar is used as part of an everyday balanced diet. I was talking to a friend from Ecuador yesterday. When Lana moved to the UK with her children she couldn't understand why people seemed so afraid of sugar, which was used quite freely and naturally in Ecuador. It is much the same as the use of MSG in China and Japan. In these countries they use everything in moderation, eat smaller amounts, often use fresh ingredients, and the children are not subjected to chemical cocktails and uncontrolled snacking.

Another thing I often observe is that people who take sugar in their drinks are often relatively slim. It's as though they use the sugar as a means of keeping their blood sugars level till the next meal, rather than opting for biscuits or cake. I don't take sugar in drinks normally, but recently I've noticed that if I go shopping a sachet of sugar in my coffee seems to help me cope till the next meal. Historically, it would have been a piece of carrot cake persuading myself it was one of my 'five a day'.

So – sugar or sweeteners? At the risk of being vilified by dentists rightfully worried about teeth, and nutritionists worried about too many chemicals for children, I feel that it would be great if we can bring the next generation up with the good old adage of 'everything in moderation.' We need to educate them to enjoy sweets and sweetened food/drink as an occasional treat – perhaps we need to look at naturally slim people and take a leaf out of their book – and we need to shop wisely regarding foods such as cereals which can be loaded with sugar.

These days it's easy to check the sugar content on a product – the higher on the list the greater percentage of sugar in the product. My real concern is all the 'no added sugar' products available now, which often contain aspartame and acesulfame K which historically were only for the 'slimming trade'. We're now bringing children up on dubious additives, putting them on a 'diet' from a very young age, and effectively bringing them up on a drug that was first formulated to treat people with ulcers (aspartame).

If you want to use a sweetener instead of sugar in you or your child's drinks, sucralose products may be the best option which some supermarket brands are now using. (Sucralose is derived from adding chlorine atoms to sugar molecules resulting in a substance 600 times sweeter than sugar, but is one eighth of the calorific value to sugar). However, even this should be used in moderation.

It's vital that we as a generation start to get this right with our children, as I believe the problems we see now with health issues such as diabetes will only be the tip of the iceberg if we carry on misleading our children's tastebuds and glucose levels.

Maybe if you use drinks with added sugar, try to keep these

to meal times and introduce good old water between meals, which I know is easier said than done!

(I also need to practice what I preach regarding the use of high-sugar foods).

E211 Sodium Benzoate

What is it?
Sodium benzoate a preservative.

Where is it used?
Sodium benzoate is found in some products such as soft drinks, sauces, medicines and toiletries (especially bath products – even famous brand baby bath).

Although some acidic food products and spices (apples, plums, cinnamon) naturally contain sodium benzoate, it is often added as a preservative to squashes, fizzy drinks, sauces, ice pops, It is also used to prevent fermentation in wine.

Sodium benzoate is banned from food and drink products designed for children under 3. However it is prolific in their toiletries, especially bath products (even famous brand baby bath). My personal theory is trials on this additive have been inconclusive, as bath products and children bathing in them have not been included. I believe this product can be ingested through the skin similar to things like nicotine patches/hormone treatments.

Is it known by any other name?
Benzoate of soda.

Mark's story, written with information from Sue, his mum

'WHAT'S IN CARBONARA?'

In a broad Midlands accent, a desperate phone call from Sue a few weeks ago.

'Nothing, it should be fine' was my reply. 'But what did Mark have to drink?'

'Lemonade.'

'Would that be lemonade on tap then?' I ask. 'It probably had sodium benzoate in.'

Mark had been out to a pub restaurant for lunch with his college, and by the evening he was hyperactive and difficult to control. Sue had had to physically restrain him in his room.

I met Sue and Mark at a Gym club 6 yrs ago, that I took Tony, our foster boy to. She mentioned about Mark's behavioural problems and mood swings etc, and guess what I mentioned my food additive theory, and gave her the yellow card.

At the time Sue didn't tell me much about Mark's history, and I had assumed his problems had been more aggression and mood swings rather than anything else. Over the years we've become friends as fellow 'parents' of young lads with special needs, regular catch ups on the phone, and the odd social occasion.

I knew Mark was a lot better and coping with life and school well, and I was also aware Mark was starting to do very well in sport. But there had been other pressing family issues that Paul and I were able to support Sue with, so Mark's past did not 'crop up' until I asked them if I could use their story in my book. In some ways I'm struggling to write this as I just think people will think this is just too good to be true, but it is!

Sue and Mark had moved to Sussex from the Midlands

in 2002. Mark, now 19, was born with a type of cerebral palsy, and at the age of seven was diagnosed with Worcester Drought syndrome. At the time there were only 250 other cases recorded in the world. Mark's early years proved to be a testing time for Sue, as Mark not only needed a succession of physiotherapy and splints to enable him to walk, he had epilepsy which was also diagnosed at the age of seven after 18 months of many tests and hospital visits.

He was extremely hyperactive most of the time – on one occasion he picked a television up over his head and threw it against the wall. He was also a very sore loser, and also prone to falling a lot, which resulted in him having to wear a helmet all the time. If that wasn't enough he was in nappies till the age of 11.

Sue felt that Mark's behaviour did improve slightly when they moved to Sussex – the school he'd been attending in the Midlands used to give the children sweets and chocolate (this would have been before the voluntary ban on the four worst food colours). He also used to have a lot of cartons of the famous blackcurrant drink (which at that time would have had sodium benzoate in), and was 'hooked' on famous brand cheesy snacks which contain MSG, and could eat six bags at a time.

On moving to Sussex Sue tried to cut down the amount of sweets and snacks Mark had. She'd also taken note of how the physiotherapists had worked with him and consistently carried on his therapy herself. When she met me she had been trying a gluten-free diet that had been recommended to her, but she didn't feel it made much difference. Sue started to avoid the food additives on my yellow card, and within a few days she saw a difference in Mark. He started to be a lot calmer and more loving, and she was even able to sit and read with him. Over the last few years not only has Mark's behaviour completely changed, he hasn't had an epileptic seizure since Sue stopped using the dubious additives. On a trip back to her sons in the Midlands, none of the family could believe the change in him.

Mark attended a special needs senior school where sport was greatly encouraged. He started to become very good at running (which was something he could not tolerate at one time), and enjoyed going to competitions and events with the school team. In Windsor in 2010 he was spotted by a scout for the Paralympics team. Mark has just under 400 gold, silver and bronze medals and many certificates. He narrowly missed selection for the 2012 Paralympics, but is now looking forward to Rio 2016. He's very much a 'winner' in my book.

As with the 'carbonara' incident there are 'blips' with Marks behaviour. Mark is now at college doing a 'life skills' course. They go out for lunch once a week, and if they go to a carvery and have the gravy (catering gravy nearly always has MSG in) or anywhere that does the 'on tap' drinks (which still have sodium benzoate in) Sue gets an evening of, at best, hyperactivity. At worst he has to be restrained to stop him trashing his room.

Mark is starting to be 'aware' of what he needs to avoid regarding the rogue additives, but it isn't always easy for him as his reading isn't that good, and finds it difficult to advocate for himself. College staff working with him do not always understand the implications.

Why/how does sodium benzoate cause a problem?

According to research, published in 2007 by the FSA (Food

Standards Association), sodium benzoate is believed to be among the causes of children's hyperactivity. It is considered to be safe if it is consumed in small doses, which is why its concentration in food products is restricted in many countries by the food authorities.

One very important thing to take into account is that it has been reported that when sodium benzoate is mixed with other food additives, such as potassium benzoate or ascorbic acid (vitamin C), it produces benzene, which is known to be a carcinogen (causes cancer). Sodium benzoate has not been found to be a carcinogen when used on its own.

Some health complications caused by this food additive do not require medical treatment. But there is mounting evidence that there are health conditions, which require urgent medical help, including difficulty or rapid breathing, disorientation, swelling of the belly, legs or arms, gastrointestinal disorders (diarrhoea, vomiting, nausea, abdominal pain) etc.

However, these are assumptions that have yet to be proven, research is being conducted to identify whether sodium benzoate causes potentially dangerous health conditions or not. That is why it is up to you to decide whether to buy products with sodium benzoate in.

How can behaviour be improved through avoiding sodium benzoate?

Some of the parents that have changed the bath products report that their children/babies were sleeping better, and general results regarding behavioural patterns with children avoiding the additives were more consistent.

How can I avoid sodium benzoate?

- Check the label!

- Remember that sodium benzoate is found in many shower gels, bubble baths (even baby products), and some lotions etc and can be absorbed through the skin, so don't just look at food labels.

- Sodium benzoate is contained in some medications. If you need to undergo medical treatment, it may be an idea to check with your doctor the ingredient list of your medication prescribed for you or your child.

- The 'on tap' fizzy drinks in food outlets pubs and bars tend to have sodium benzoate in even if the branded version in the tin or bottle does not.

- Sodium benzoate can be mainly found in drinks and sauces, but its use in these products does seem to be in decline.

CHAPTER FIVE

Good Foods for Good Behaviour

It goes without saying that a healthy diet includes eating as many portions of fruit and vegetables per day that you can. But you may find that children who have an intolerance to certain additives often crave the very foods that contain them. Once you are more 'in control' of your child's behaviour, and they are more compliant, you will feel more empowered to resist the pressure to allow them to eat just what they like. You'll then hopefully be able to introduce healthier foods and snacks they will enjoy!

The importance of breakfast

One of the really interesting things I've discovered over the years is that children who may be intolerant to certain food additives can also suffer from low blood sugar if they do not eat/drink on a regular basis. This can result in the kind of negative behaviour we've seen throughout this book, and is even more easily avoided than the additives!

If you think about it, tea time to morning is a really long time, and blood sugar will dip overnight. Because of this it's really important children have something for breakfast to get them going. Many primary schools now have fruit options at morning break, or you may need to arrange for your child to have a snack mid-morning. They'll need this even if they've had a good breakfast, so if their lunch-time is later than 12.30pm their blood sugar levels can be kept on an even keel.

On non-school days breakfast can become a lot later than normal, especially at the weekend. So if your child seems to be a problem first thing in the morning it may be an idea to look at how they are 20 minutes after eating. If they are calmer and more able to conform maybe you'll need to keep breakfast time relatively early.

After-school snacks
Younger children may need a snack ready for them when they come out of school, or soon after you get home. The little edam-type cheeses are good but expensive, so a small chunk of cheese wrapped in foil is just as good, or something like a little box or bag of raisins. If the snack is to be at home maybe carrot, cucumber, pepper or non MSG mini rice cakes or mini bread sticks with flavoured Mayo 'dippy' (see recipes). With biscuits and non-MSG crisps/snacks try and avoid giving these every day if you can. But once a day when you are 'in control' of what they are eating is probably better than children having snacks to just keep them 'happy'.

I know some parents don't like their children having snacks after school for fear of spoiling their dinner, but if a child has their lunch at mid-day, and then doesn't eat for more than four hours after an active day, they're more likely to kick off and be in too much of a state to approach mealtime in a positive way.

The important thing is to try and avoid giving a snack after a meal if the child hasn't eaten much of the meal (easier said than done).

If your child has been affected by behavioural problems and/or mood swings caused by certain food additives, all of the above might have been very difficult to put in place. A packet of crisps might have been the only way to please or even feed your child. But hopefully if your child responds well when you try avoiding the dubious additives they will become more compliant and easier at meal times. It is great to get them to 'help' prepare food and this will hopefully encourage them try new tastes etc.

Coping with fussy eaters

Food is not just fuel. It's an important part of family and social life. A child needs to see how other people eat and see them enjoying food. If you have just one child and you eat later when they have gone to bed, how will they learn the social side of eating?

From the outset make sure a child experiences a calm happy occasion when eating. If they relate this time to mum or dad getting stressed and getting cross with them, they may use refusing food as a way of getting their own way.

When young children start eating independently, cut the food down to half of what you think should be on the plate in front of them (especially when they start to feed themselves). Then you can praise them for eating it all and give more if needed. Maybe have the dish of food on the table that you serve the child from. When children start wanting to feed themselves apparently they prefer to have finger food so carrots, potato, sweet potato and parsnips could be cooked in long chunks for instance.

Tony (our long term foster child who is now an adult) has autism, so part of his condition is being 'fussy' with food. It is often about texture, so I use the disguising vegetables idea in Chapter Seven a lot, and little does he know a shepherd's pie can have as many as seven vegetables in.

I also make him the flavoured dips (with the mayo dippy) with carrot and peppers cut into strips. Fruit is very difficult. He won't eat apples on their own, but will eat toffee apples, so they are a once or twice a week treat. He'll also eat bananas, but only in a toasted sandwich with a little brown sugar.

I also find if I make a risotto and dice peppers, onion and mushrooms well and add diced bacon at the end he will enjoy that.

When I make pizzas with the scone base I make sure I use plenty of tomato puree and place the chopped veg under the grated cheese before baking.

I peel and chop root vegetables such as potato, parsnip, swede, celeriac and carrot, boil them in either water or stock, and when cooked through drain and mash really well. Then I make the mixture into fish-cake shapes and fry in a little oil till golden brown and warmed through. Serve instead of potato, pasta or chips. A good non-stick frying pan is useful for this.

When making mashed potato I sometimes cut the potatoes quite small to boil and add some of the white part of a cauliflower, or some peeled and chopped celeriac. When cooked through drain and mash well, adding milk and butter if desired.

There are lots of other foody tips in Chapter Seven. However, if the fussiness continues, and you don't feel your child is eating from all the food groups, I'd advise talking to your doctor to see if a referral to a nutritionist or dietician is needed.

Something good to add to your family's diet – OMEGA 3

What is it?
Omega 3 and another group called omega 6 belong to a family of fats known as essential fatty acids.

Where is it found?
Oily fish, flax seeds, nuts omega 3 supplements.

Is it known by any other name?
Fish oil.

Why/how does omega 3 work?
It plays a role in virtually every cell of our body. It particularly helps brain function and co-ordination, and high doses are considered by some experts as good as or better than Ritalin, one of the drugs used for the treatment of ADHD.

How can behaviour be improved through eating omega 3 or using supplements?
There are several studies and trials that have taken place. One, which was lead by Dr Madeleine Portwood, a senior educational psychologist, described the results as 'stunning'.

The trial focused on a group of twenty disruptive young people aged between 12 and 15 from Greenfield Community Arts college, County Durham. Nineteen were considered to have moderate to severe ADHD, nineteen were also judged to have short attention spans and eighteen were also highly impulsive. At the end of the twelve-week trial – which used supplements – the number showing symptoms of ADHD had dropped to six, only three were severely inattentive, and only six highly impulsive. The supplements were Eye Q smooth, a blend of omega 3 and omega 6 by Equazen.

How can I add omega 3 to my family's diet?
By using oily fish such as salmon (the packs of budget off-cuts of smoked salmon are good) mackerel, tuna, herring, pilchards

and sardines. If your family find it difficult to eat fish there is a vast array of omega 3 supplements now, and a large retail chemist has 'buy two get one free' offers all the time. You can buy capsule or liquid form and even chewy bear type sweets with it in. If you start an omega 3 supplement you need to carry on using it on a long term basis, as the beneficial effects will wear off if you stop using it.

Heidi's story

I met Heidi and her husband, who was an Australian called Simon, several years ago when she only had one child a boy called Kurt. My friend and I were using her bed and breakfast in Switzerland. We loved it so much we returned several times over a five-year period. During that time Heidi had another child, Freddie, so it was lovely for us to see the boys growing up.

Freddie was about 2 by the time of our last visit, and had been having tantrums and mood swings for no reason at all. This was starting to get very tiring and worrying for Heidi, as Kurt also was prone to unexplained mood swings and the boys found it difficult to play together.

I mentioned about food additives to Heidi, and she was keen to follow my idea. But I was also aware that in Switzerland there seemed to be far more MSG in certain foods, and even in a seasoning you find on most Swiss restaurant tables (my first couple of visits to Switzerland in another area were marred by my mood swings until I worked out that I needed to avoid the MSG where possible). But the Swiss don't have as many snacks and drinks with the other additives in, and Swiss culture (as with the Chinese and Japanese) expects children to behave.

Also, Swiss children go home at lunch time for two hours, so there are no 'lunch-box' cocktails of additives.

I suggested as the boys didn't like fish that an omega 3 supplement might be good for them. A few months later I emailed Heidi to see how they were doing, and this is the email I got back:

We changed (almost all) the food in our kitchen. That was not easy, I was really surprised that that mononatriumglutamat (E621) is in almost everything.

But I am in a good way and found everything without it in different brands, just one thing I could not find yet. I think it's called Gravy in English? I want to go down to Interlaken and have a look there. It took me quite a while to get organized again and I am really happy that Simon (her husband) 'jumped on' as well. Otherwise it would not work.

I did also started buying omega 3 Fish oil (specially for kids) and I am happy that Kurt takes it well. Unfortunately its just for kids older than 5, but I do also try to cook more fish. Freddy is eating it, just Kurt won't.

Judy, I guess you won't be very surprised if I tell you that I slowly can see a change in my kid. I was a bit sceptical. Freddy doesn't scream anymore like he used to. If he's doing something that he's not allowed to do and I tell him off, he goes to his room and closes the door behind him, and comes back when he is happy again. Kurt is pretty good as well, he does still have his angry moments but it is ok. And I guess, I am much more relaxed as well.

JUDY, THANKS A LOT!

CHAPTER SIX

Unlearning Negative Behaviour

Some may say that if parents/carers were to follow the positive behaviour strategies I mention below a child could well start behaving/conforming without worrying about food additives. For some it may be true, but in my experience (and many others') a child will find it so much easier to be consistently 'good' and conform as others expect them to when they avoid the additives.

Of course if a child has a specific learning difficulty they may not conform through no fault of their own as people may expect/hope. However, by avoiding the dubious additives the outcome of their behaviour may well be a great deal better, helping them to cope with life and different situations.

The benefits of starting early

It's great that in the last few years I've co-run a toddler group, because the younger a child is when a parent tries avoiding the dubious additives, the better the outcome for the future for the child, and there will probably be fewer behavioural problems to 'unlearn'. However many children of different ages, and some teenagers/adults, have also had pleasing results.

You may have heard the term 'self-fulfilling prophesy'. In basic terms this means a child will act and be like he or she has been told/heard they are, for instance if every time a child goes out with adults and they hear 's/he is very shy' rather than 's/he just takes time to get used to people' that child could end up being very shy. If s/he hears 's/he is a pain in the neck and just does not do what I say' s/he could well grow up to be and do just that!

How to give praise
A very young child may not know when they are behaving as expected or not, but could be very used to people telling him to be good, behave, and don't do that.

If you try avoiding the additives you should hopefully see a difference in just a few days, but you will need to give your child constant cues to when they are doing as they should such as:

- 'that's good that you played nicely on that seesaw'

- 'that's really good that you sat and did that drawing'

- 'that was really good that you sat still to eat your lunch'

- 'I'm really pleased you did not make a fuss when I said you could not have another biscuit before dinner'

'It's as though you are giving them permission to behave!'

Remember!
Body language and facial expression are important, you can show a child you are pleased with them without saying a word.

Teaching children to be part of the crowd

If you try avoiding the additives with an older child and they start to conform/behave better they may well 'blend' into normality with his peers and siblings. It can be easy to forget to praise your child and say you are pleased with them, and you like how they are behaving.

Some children who have had severe behaviour problems will have never had much praise because they have not done anything to get it, children are very sensitive and can crave praise and approval from their parents/care-givers.

Another good strategy for children is for them to hear you telling other people how pleased you are with them, as though you do not know they can 'hear' you.

Involving other adults

You will also need to get other adults in their lives to do the same, and get them to believe in your child, to enforce the message.

For older children in school, other children (and even teachers and school staff sometimes) may still expect your child to play up, it's important to get the teachers and assistants on side and clued up to what is happening, but maybe leave telling them for a couple of weeks until your child has had the chance to see if avoiding the additives help, if it does the teacher may well have noticed already when you tell them.

Some parents/carers choose not to tell their child that they are avoiding certain additives at first which is easy to do as it is usually just changing a brand. This way a child would not feel a failure in the unlikely event that avoiding certain additives made no difference at all.

A 16 year old boy with special needs came to live with us.

After six weeks I went to his open evening, and the teacher asked what we had done to him. I had been unaware that he had been previously very aggressive at times in school and had a very short attention span. This wasn't happening now, and he was able to stay 'on task' for more than 20 minutes at a time, which did not happen before. I did have to ask the school canteen to avoid these additives for his food too, you sometimes need a 'diplomatic hat' in these situations.

Older children
When an older child is on board about the additives, you may well need to do some 'repair' work with them. This means talking through how other people saw them, how they can show that they are able to behave and how to cope with other children who knew how to 'press' their buttons.

• Teach the child the kind of body language to show that they're 'not bovvered.'

• Children can learn to say things to themselves, like 'am I bovvered' or 'whatever' and not say them out loud.

• Maybe invite other children to tea who you might not have been able to do before, to give your child a chance to show their 'different' side.

Benefits for all
If you avoid the additives with yourself and all the family, you may well find an added bonus, you and others may also have been affected in some way, so you will find you are able to cope with life a bit better and have more patience to say the least.

CHAPTER SEVEN

Everyday Recipe Tips

I have put some ideas, food tips together that will hopefully help, especially if you have fussy eaters to feed. If you're on a limited income, most of the ingredients I use can also be selected from supermarket basic/budget range (even mixed herbs and stock cubes). It goes without saying all the ingredients I use can be found without any of the dubious list of additives – but remember to always check the label initially just in case!

Amounts are approximate and you can vary them if you need to.

Tools
A hand blender is a really useful gadget. You can buy them for a few pounds from some supermarkets. If you use a hand blender make sure you blend in a high sided container/saucepan or you might 'pebble dash' the kitchen.

You can also use a jug blender, smoothie maker or a food processor, but a hand blender is easiest to wash up.

A cheese slicer or potato peeler is useful to thinly slice cheese as some children do not like the texture.

Budget-minded foody tips

- When using vegetable/olive oil for frying or roasting veg in the oven use just 5ml per person (level 5ml medicine spoon) so although you are frying or roasting you are not using too much oil.

- Basic/budget/value fruit and veg can be very good, and if you buy it whole it's much cheaper than buying it ready prepared.

- When buying items like sauces, it's always an idea to check that the sugar and salt content aren't higher in the budget brands than the more expensive ones.

- When cooking minced meat for a shepherds pie or a Bolognese, keep the sauce fairly liquid and add porridge oats to thicken and add bulk. If you use a jar of sauce you can always add a little extra water.

- A little sugar added to tomato based sauces can bring out the flavour.

- Add cooked/tinned lentils or porridge oats to minced meat dishes to make it go further.

- When using minced meat for Burgers or meatballs add stuffing mix made up.

- Chop half a pack of budget bacon off-cuts and add ten minutes before the end of cooking an onion and mushroom risotto.

- Packet mashed potato is a good standby, when you have

made it up you can add either wholegrain mustard, horseradish sauce and/or grated cheese.

- Tinned ravioli placed in dish with grated cheese on top and baked in the oven makes a quick tasty meal.

- When having jacket potatoes, for a low-fat option instead of butter or margarine I use either mint sauce or horseradish sauce.

When stir-frying veg (children will often eat beanshoots) add some soy sauce near the end of cooking to flavour it (not suitable for very young children because of the salt content).

Basic/budget/value pizzas are OK but light on cheese, so add extra grated or sliced cheese. If you put finely diced peppers, ham or salami on too, make sure the cheese covers the bits for the 'fussy eaters.'

For 'pizza rolls' cut a roll in half, spread with tomato puree add chopped veg and/or meat if desired. Top with grated cheese and bake in the oven for about 7-10 minutes. You can also do this with baguettes cut in half.

When cooking sausages in the oven cut them lengthways but not right through. They'll open out when cooking, children like them and they take less time to cook.

Some children don't like sausage skins, so I sometimes take them off and reshape the sausages into burger shapes (two per burger), then either cook in the oven or fry in a little oil.

If you have a busy day and want to do the likes of fish fingers, nuggets, burgers for tea, maybe try adding the mayonnaise dippy and sticks of veg or do the vedgy wedges.

Or just have tinned baked beans or tinned spaghetti maybe with a little grated cheese on.

Disguising vegetables
Children and teenagers alike can be very fussy when it comes to vegetables so disguising them is one way to go. Here are is one of the best ways I know to add them to your family's diet:

Basic (no bits) soup base sauce
This is a brilliant way of hiding vegetables and can be used in several different ways just by adding different flavouring.

Ingredients:
- 300g **vegetables** (choose a mixture of at least two of these veg: carrots, leeks, courgette, celery, celeriac, swede, peppers, butternut squash) peeled and chopped.

- 1 medium **onion**, peeled and sliced.

- 1 veg/beef/chicken/lamb **stock cube** or one of the new stock pots (If you're making this for younger children only use half a stock cube, a low salt version, or leave it out altogether. Maybe add extra herbs).

- 450 ml **water**

Method:
1. Put the water and stock cube in a pan with the onion and vegetables.

2. Bring to the boil then reduce to a simmer for about 10-15minutes until vegetables are tender.

3. When the ingredients have slightly cooled blend ingredients with a hand blender, and season as desired.

This basic soup sauce can now be used several ways:

Add some of the 'soup' to the tomato base when making a **Bolognese** sauce. This can make it go further, adding some tomato puree will make it richer.

To make a 'no bits' **Shepherds Pie** add some of the 'soup' to your mince and add some gravy granules to thicken. Top with potato and sweet potato (if desired) mashed.

When making a **curry** flavour your basic 'soup mix' with curry paste or powder of your choice and add to your meat and stir fried veg as required, add tomato puree for a richer flavour.

To make **meatballs** use minced meat of your choice and add made up stuffing mix to make the meat go further you can also add an egg. For the sauce use some of the 'soup mix' and add passata, tinned tomato or tomato puree, and herbs of your choice.

Winning ways with potatoes

Use up mashed potato by adding some flour and egg to make a stiff pancake mixture and make potato pancakes (about scotch pancake size) serve with tomato or brown sauce. If there is wheat intolerance you can just use the potato and egg, but add salt for flavour.

Wedges

Ingredients:
- 1 or 2 **potatoes** per person (depending on the size)

- 5ml tsp **vegetable or olive oil** per person

- Optional flavourings:
  Crushed/paste or Garlic salt, Chinese five spice or celery salt.

Method:
1. Wash and cut your potatoes into wedge shapes (very chunky chip size).
2. Put the oil into a large bowl with any flavourings you're using.
3. Stir the wedges into the oil until they're covered.
4. Tip them onto a baking tray that has either non stick greaseproof paper, non stick foil, or a Teflon baking sheet, making sure you only have one layer of wedges.
5. Bake on the highest setting of your oven for 20 minutes then reduce the heat to 350F, 180C, Gas 4 for about 15-20mins depending on size, until wedges are golden brown and cooked through.

Variations:
- This works just as well for peeled wedges of sweet potatoes, parsnips or swede.
- I also sometimes add a small peeled onion for each person that likes them.
- I also do my roast potatoes in the same way but cook them a bit longer.

Jacket potatoes

When doing jacket potatoes in the oven bake enough for two for each person, so one day you have jacket potatoes, the next day you could do one of the following.

- Slice thickly and fry in a little oil or even spray oil, until crisp and golden each side for delicious fried potato. Great with a cooked breakfast.

- Cut them in quarter's length ways lay them on a non stick baking sheet or tray and brush or spray them with oil, then grill or bake them till golden brown in a high oven for chunky jacket wedges.

- Cut the cold jacket potatoes in half length ways and scoop contents into a bowl. Keeping the skins to one side, add about 25g of grated cheese per potato and some finely chopped onion (you can pre-cook onion if preferred or omit altogether) you could add freshly chopped chives (or dried chives) and use spring onion instead of onion. Mix all ingredients well together and place mixture into the potato skins bake in a hot oven for 15 minutes or place under a hot grill until piping hot right through.

- For a lower-fat stuffed jacket potato use a 120g pack of basics/budget/value smoked salmon trimmings (enough for four potatoes) to mix in the potato as above and bake/grill until completely heated through. You could add dried/fresh fennel or tarragon to taste.

Mayonnaise 'dippies'

The shops now do a wide range of flavoured mayonnaise, but

you can easily make your own with a jar of mayonnaise (budget /basics/value if needed). The flavoured mayonnaise can be used as dips with veg/salad or mini bread sticks, or as part of the filling in sandwiches, rolls, pitas, wraps, bagels.

Place the required amount in a bowl you can then add one of the following:

Mint sauce: minty mayo is great with tinned tuna mixed in, or diced lamb if you're feeling flash. Also nice with carrot, cucumber, sliced peppers or sweet potato sticks as a snack.

Horseradish sauce: horseradish mayo is nice with cold beef and salad, hardboiled eggs or as a dip as above.

Garlic: add crushed fresh/dried/or paste in tubes, use as a dip, or add diced chicken and sweet corn.

Tomato sauce: makes a seafood type sauce a nice dip with Scampi, fish fingers, prawns/prawn cocktail.

Whole grain or ordinary mustard: good with cold meats/sausages.

Curry powder or paste: good with cold meats and in wraps.

Sweet Chilli sauce: good with bread sticks crisp etc.

Desserts

- Make up a block of jelly with half the water when cool add a large pot of natural yoghurt or a tin of custard blend together and set in individual pots or a bowl then you have creamy yoghurt type desserts.

- Make up a block of jelly with half the water then blend in a blender with either tinned or stewed fruit such as tinned oranges, rhubarb, apple, apricots, peaches, pears. Place in a bowl or individual pots to set.

- Pierce a banana then place in the microwave till it goes brown all over, place the banana in a bowl slit the side open and serve with cream or ice cream or turn the cooked flesh into a bowl and mix well with yoghurt or custard.

- Frozen fruits are fun such as peeled frozen bananas, stoned cherries, grapes, blueberries. Do ensure you defrost the fruits slightly before serving.

Breakfasts

For a quick ready breakfast soak overnight about 35g of porridge oats per person in a fruit yoghurt with a little milk added. Then add your favourite fruit chopped up such as tinned apricots, cherries, strawberries, raspberries, blueberries, a few raisins or sultanas. Frozen fruits are good too such as forest fruits or cherries. If adding apple banana or pear put them into the oat mixture just before you eat it, or the fruit goes brown.

There is now an array of flavoured ready mix breakfast porridge, it is just as easy to make you own and much cheaper. Make your porridge as instructed on packet add sugar as desired then add:

- A chopped or grated banana

- A grated apple with cinnamon

- Half a teaspoon of cinnamon and a few raisins

- A few fresh or frozen blueberries

- When making up the porridge add a tablespoon full of hot chocolate powder per person for chocolate porridge. Try without added sugar first or use cocoa and add sugar.

- A few chocolate chips for an occasional treat

- Golden syrup or honey instead of the sugar

Eggy bread
Beat an egg with a little milk add a little salt to taste dip half slices of bread in the mix lift out and then fry in a little preheated hot oil in a pan, till golden brown each side serve with tomato/brown sauce or even a little jam spread on it.

Eating out and about
Eating out can be a bit of a minefield when you are trying to avoid certain food additives, so I've included a few pointers and information here that might help you. Once you get to know what you can and can't have, and which places are the 'safest' to eat at, it does get easier.

Avoiding all the dubious additives all the time is virtually impossible, but if you can avoid having a cocktail and maybe just one thing with an additive in, the outcome might be more manageable. For instance, if you decide to have the gravy, avoid the 'on tap' fizzy as well.

- A lot of pubs/restaurants/major food outlets have the 'on tap' fizzy drinks. As far as I'm aware most contain sodium benzoate, used as a preservative in the syrup mixes, etc. Many also contain aspartame as well – even if the product is not diet and the bottled/canned variety is ok to buy. Also watch the individual size bottled famous brand fruit squashes and milk shakes, which again can contain sodium benzoate and/or aspartame or acesulfame K. Ask staff to check the labels of the bulk mixes for the milkshakes – but it's probably best to ask when they're not too busy.

- It's good to gather your own list of alternative drinks children can have when you are out, such as fruit juices, bottled fruit juice mixes, bottled non-diet colas and sparkling water.

- If you're going to a carvery there's always gravy, and most tend to use the famous brand variety which contains MSG. Why not take a little pot or bag of your own granules, and ask if the gravy has MSG in (including the stock). If the answer's yes, ask for some of your gravy to be made up in a jug or cup.

- With burger establishments the well known brand burgers are OK, but some of the nugget and fish finger coatings may have MSG in. The famous coated chicken is heavily flavoured with MSG. You also need to watch the on tap drinks/milk shakes and some of the sauces.

- With Chinese food some restaurants now advertise the fact that they don't use added MSG in their menus/ products . If you ask you won't be the first!

- Fish and chips are ok, but watch the sausages and meat pies in chip shops as some have MSG in. Also if you order burgers from them it may be best to get them to check.

- Full English breakfasts – you may need to check the sausages but the rest should be ok.

- Pizzas are usually OK, but just watch the ones that have processed/salami type meats on for the MSG. Again, beware the 'on tap' fizzy drinks.

- On a healthy note fast foods can be fine if used as an occasional special treat also some do healthier option 'extras' such as bags of ready prepared fruit etc.

Natalie's email

Natalie was a trainee social worker, on placement with the agency we work for. I got to know her well as she did our supervision, and we met on several occasions. After the first couple of sessions I could see she had problems with headaches and mood swings, but it took me a while to persuade her to try my ideas for a couple of weeks which she finally did.

Hi Judy

I just wanted to take a moment to let you know how I have been getting on since you discussed with me the effects of the additives such as MSG and aspartame in some of the everyday foods that we purchase.

Initially I was a little sceptical and thought it would not work and could not possible make such a difference to my life. I also thought it could turn out to be a nuisance looking at all the foods to see if it contained these products. However the purse-sized cards you gave me with the brief but essential information on were extremely useful.

I am not sure if you remember me explaining how I suffered with severe headaches and have realised over recent years how very abrupt and snappy I can be, especially in the mornings. This behaviour of mine has had a massive impact on my everyday life, including my marriage breaking down after 5 years. I was not the easiest person to live with and how my children coped with my moods I have no idea. Everyone that knew me would laugh and joke about how they was no way you could have a conversation with me in the mornings because my moods were so bad, even my young children learnt not to speak to me.

After a few conversations with yourself and your advice about these additives I decided would it really hurt to try and see if it made any difference. Also because I am in my third year of University and this has been a very stressful year with juggling everything I needed to try something.

One of the easiest things to change was to stop buying certain brands of gravy and crisps that I loved, after realising it was not about cutting out the foods completely but rather finding an alternate product that did not contain the MSG or aspartame it became easy and was no hassle to when I purchased my weekly shop.

I have found the outcomes of recent months have been

that I have not been suffering with the severe headaches that I was previously, even with having to sit at a computer all day every day. My mother and my children and many others have commented at how I have apparently 'lightened up' so much and these people were not aware at the time of what I was doing. I feel in myself much calmer and more relaxed, even as a third year student who should be stressed out!!

Another a aspect was my monthly periods, well I was hell to live with and always used pmt as an excuse to my behaviour, but now I sail through my monthly periods with ease and it is unbelievable. I now do not have to dread my periods because I manage.

The biggest thing for me is that a few months ago I started a new relationship and this is going from strength to strength. Previously the smallest thing would have annoyed me but now I find I can discuss things in a calm and manageable way and my relationship is the best I have ever experienced and I am aware this is down to my moods changing and for not feeling so stressed out. When I try to explain this people I wonder if they think I am making it up, even my mum and friends who have seen such a change in me. All I can say is that everyone should try this because until you do you cannot really understand the impact it has on you.

I would like to thank you massively for the advice you gave and shared with me and for helping me to change a lifetime habit.

I am sure that my kids have also benefited from the change in products that we use because my son who is going through his GCSE is doing so with such ease, and yet last year with his mock exams he was very stressed.

Again thank you so much, and it would be a pleasure to keep in touch and be updated with any new information that you may have.

Best wishes

Natalie

Recent update from Natalie

Natalie emailed me recently to let me know she was continuing to do well avoiding the dubious additive. However, she had twice fallen out with her new boyfriend but on both occasions he had cooked her a meal. Natalie had checked what he was using for gravy granules and 'bingo' the famous brand variety. Her man has changed his granules, and the relationship is growing strong!

CHAPTER EIGHT

What Next?

I hope this book has inspired you to at least try avoiding the dubious food additives for a couple of weeks or so. I know some of the stories seem too good to be true – but they are!

You should have seen by now that these additives really do seem to affect some people's health and behaviour. And if it works for the people I come into contact with in my little corner of West Sussex, imagine the amazing results we could have across the country!

It's my dearest wish that you'll get pleasing results by avoiding them, and that you'll have a sense of relief at finding the cause of a behavioural problem or maybe even a health condition. But be warned you will also feel angry that these additives are allowed to be in food and drink when they can cause so much harm and distress to some.

Over to you

In my book I have just given you a 'flavour' of how powerful and controlling the food industry is today. So how can we bring about change so that people don't have to look at everything they are consuming?

1. If you try avoiding the additives mentioned in this book PLEASE PLEASE let me have your feedback (positive and negative) using the email address on The Additive Puzzle website **www.additivepuzzle.co.uk**. I'll collate the information so that I can 'inform' the powers that be regarding the findings. Who knows what 'can of worms' we will open!

2. I originally set out to write a book about children's behaviour, but as you have read these additives seem to affect anyone of any age, so your stories are vital to get an overall picture. I'm particularly interested to hear from people who feel they may be addicted the famous brand diet colas. Maybe you'll be contributing to my next book!

3. If enough people stop buying products containing the dubious additives, the manufacturers will have to change their ways.

4. Mention this book to others – it could be the best Christmas present ever for someone you really care about.

Index

Useful Links and Further Reading

I deliberately kept my book 'basic' and 'user friendly' for parents and individuals with the hope that people will feel able to at least try and avoid the worst additives in their food and drink. However, there are of course many other additives that may be dubious.

If you wish to find out more about these additives there is a wealth of information and many websites out there – I've listed a few that you may find useful, and some books that may help you in your quest to eat and drink more healthily.

Books

What's Really In Your Basket? By Bill Statham published by Summersdale
A comprehensive list of food and cosmetic additives with a useful traffic lights system for highlighting ok additives and those best avoided or used in moderation.

What The Label Doesn't Tell You By Sue Dibb a co-director of the Food Commission.
Although printed in 1997 much of the information is still relevant today and is available on Amazon.

Toxic Childhood By Sue Palmer
This book contains an extensive amount of research regarding

the food industry and what they are doing to our food and drink, mixed with some effective parenting tips, but would need to be used in small bite size chunks.

The Art of Hiding Vegetables By Karen Bali and Sally Child
A good practical guide to helping your child eat more vegetables and fruit which includes 'breaking old habits and psychology'.

Websites

hacs.org.uk – website of the Hyperactive Children's Support Group, a charity founded by Sally Bunday MBE. Sally's work is more specifically targeted at children with ADHD (Attention Deficit Hyperactive Disorder).

The HACSG is Britain's leading force in advocating a dietary approach regarding ADHD, which is based on the Fiengold programme (see below) which looks to eliminate most food additives from food and drink and advocates a 1930's style diet.

MSGTruth.org – an American website regarding the effects of MSG, this is very American and very comprehensive, proceed with caution!

Sweetpoison.com – A website about Dr Janet Star Hulls work regarding Aspartame, again in American and can be frightening!

Parentlineplus.org.uk – provides help and information to help families and children in all situations.

actiononadditives.com – a campaigning group which is hoping to get six artificial colours banned from all food and from children's medicines, and further research into the use of Sodium benzoate.

foodsmatter.com – very large website which includes articles and research reports on allergy, intolerance and sensitivity, and related health problems.

netmums.co.uk – a useful resource for parents, they have an extended list of fifteen food additives to avoid.

food.gov.uk – website of the government's Food Standards Agency (FSA), whose job it is to ensure the UK's food and drink are safe. The site gives plenty of information about food additives, as well as healthy eating. Although they will advocate there is not conclusive evidence that certain additives cause behavioural/health problems.

truthinlabelling.org – has a comprehensive list of ingredients that contain naturally occurring MSG.

Further research

The Feingold Programme
As long ago as 1975 a book called *Why Your Child Is Hyperactive* was published by Dr. Feingold, an American paediatrician. His claim was that the behaviour of between 30% and 50% of hyperactive children improved dramatically if foods containing artificial colours, preservatives and flavourings, and foods

containing naturally occurring salicylvates, were removed from their diets. This has caused controversy and debate that is still ongoing today.

Isle of Wight Study

In 2002 the Food Standards Agency produced a report that gave results of research that had been conducted on a group of 100 3 year old children living on the Isle of Wight. They tested four food colours and sodium benzoate following media reports that suggested a link between hyperactivity and certain additives, and parents reported that one in four children showed significant improvement in their behaviour once the additives were withdrawn from their diet. However, scientists deemed the results inconclusive.

I believe these trials were inconclusive because the preservative sodium benzoate was probably still in the children's bath/toiletries products, and MSG and aspartame were not included in the trials.

University of Southampton tests

In 2007, results from the University of Southampton suggested that there was a link between increased hyperactivity in children and certain food colourings and the preservative sodium benzoate. The study looked at over 260 children in two age groups.

The European Food Safety Authority (EFSA) looked at the Southampton University research and decided that the results were not clear cut. EFSA were not convinced that the small alterations in attention and activity that were observed in the study would actually interfere with children's ability to think and perform schoolwork.

However, from these studies/trials and others since 2009 the UK Food Standards Agency (FSA) has asked UK food producers to voluntarily withdraw use of these colours. The foods containing these colours should contain the label, 'May have an adverse effect on activity and attention in children'. The colours are:

- sunset yellow (E110)
- quinoline yellow (E104)
- carmoisine (E122)
- allura red (E129)
- tartrazine (E102)
- ponceau 4R (E124)

With this research again just certain food colourings and sodium benzoate were tested. MSG and aspartame were not included!

Durham Trials
These looked at the positive effect of fatty acids (omega 3 fish oils) on behaviour and some learning difficulties including ADHD, dyspraxia and dyslexia.
www.durhamtrial.org

Acknowledgements

I'd like to dedicate this book to my long-suffering husband, Paul, who has supported and encouraged me in writing this book. To Andy my 'inspiration', and my family and friends who tried not to glaze over too much when I started talking about food additives.

Thank you to everyone who has tried avoiding the 'big four' so far. I'd especially like to thank those who have shared their stories/emails with me, and allowed them to be published in the hope that others may be inspired to give it a try and, hopefully, change lives. All the contributors' names have been changed.

And thank you to Sarah Palmer, my editor, for her patience and making me believe I could write a book!

These cards are just like the ones I gave people when I started getting interested in additives. Why not cut them out and keep them in your purse or wallet, so you can take them with you when you go shopping? Get them laminated and they'll last even longer.

Main food additives to try and avoid

E621 Monosodium Glutamate MSG (flavour enhancer) mainly found in some gravy granules/stock cubes/salami sticks/crisps and snacks/ Chinese and processed foods

E951 Aspartame and Acesuflame K **E950** (artificial sweeteners) found in some diet and no added sugar food/drinks

E211 Sodium Benzoate (preservative) found in some drinks/ sauces/ bubble bath and baby toiletries

www.additivepuzzle.co.uk

Main food additives to try and avoid

E621 Monosodium Glutamate MSG (flavour enhancer) mainly found in some gravy granules/stock cubes/salami sticks/crisps and snacks/ Chinese and processed foods

E951 Aspartame and Acesuflame K **E950** (artificial sweeteners) found in some diet and no added sugar food/drinks

E211 Sodium Benzoate (preservative) found in some drinks/ sauces/ bubble bath and baby toiletries

www.additivepuzzle.co.uk